I0781808

VEGETARIAN COOKBOOK FOR BEGINNERS 2024

Explore The Flavour Of Plant-based With Over 50 Recipes

Bridgette Johns

Copyright Notice for Bridgette Johns' "The Vegetarian Cookbook for Beginners 2024"

© 2024 Bridgette Johns. All rights reserved.

Title: The Vegetarian Cookbook for Beginners 2024

Author: Bridgette Johns

Publication Year: 2024

Publisher: [Publisher's Name: Martins Dorwell Books Publications LTD

Copyright Statement:

All content included in this book, such as text, graphics, logos, images, and software, is the property of Bridgette Johns or her content suppliers and is protected by United States and international copyright laws.

Unauthorized reduplication or distribution of this material is banned and may affect civil and felonious penalties. For warrants, please communicate with the author (Bridgette Johns).

Table of contents

A creamy coconut rice pudding topped with fresh mango slices.

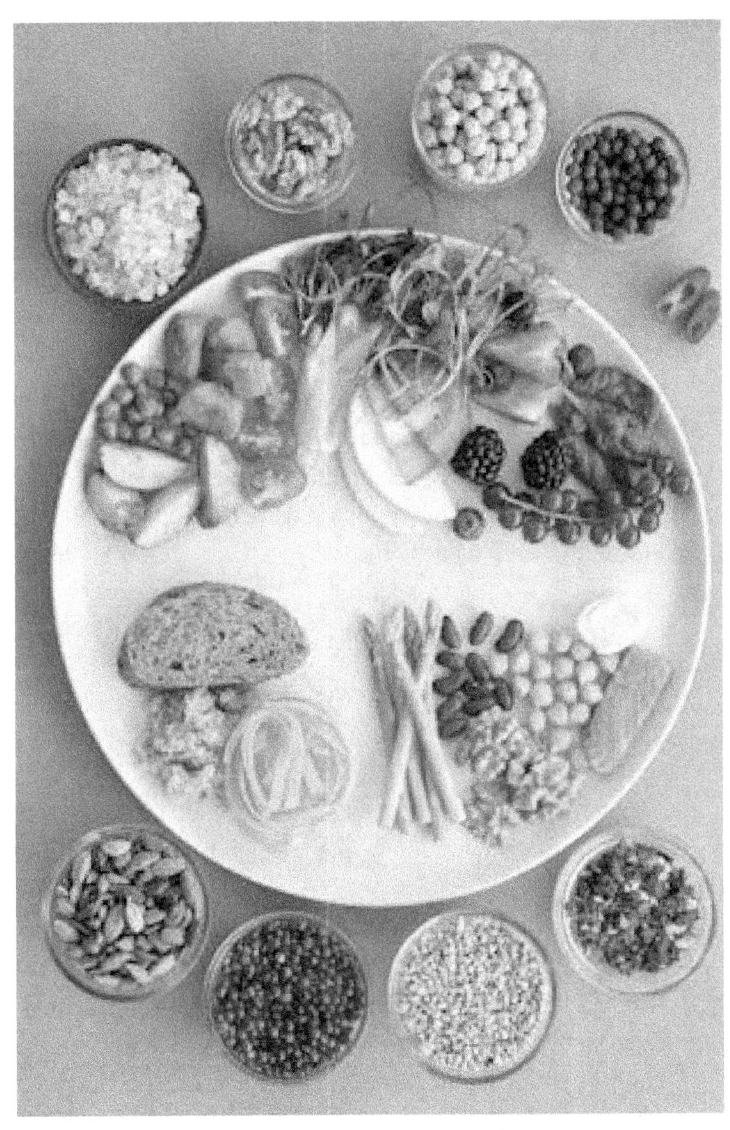

INTRODUCTION

Welcome to The Beginner's Vegetarian Cookbook!

Whether you're considering transitioning to a vegetarian lifestyle for health reasons, environmental concerns, or simply a desire to explore new culinary horizons, this cookbook is your guide to making delicious, satisfying, and nutritious vegetarian meals. Designed especially for beginners, our goal is to make your journey into vegetarianism as enjoyable and straightforward as possible

Why Choose Vegetarian?

Embark on a culinary adventure with the Vegetarian Cookbook for Beginners 2024, where vibrant health and tantalizing flavors meet in every recipe. This cookbook is not just about food; it is about transforming your lifestyle and embracing the abundant benefits of a plant-based diet.

Imagine Mary, a busy mother of two, who struggled with energy dips and meal planning chaos. With the help of this cookbook, she discovered simple, nutritious meals that her whole family loves. Now, she enjoys more energy and peace of mind knowing she is nourishing her loved ones with wholesome ingredients.

Or consider John, a college student overwhelmed by fast food options. This cookbook became his go-to guide, making it easy to whip up budget-friendly, delicious meals in minutes. His grades improved, and he felt more focused and vibrant than ever.

Each recipe is crafted to be easy, accessible, and packed with nutrients, helping you make a seamless transition to a healthier lifestyle. From hearty breakfasts to delectable dinners, this cookbook offers something for every taste and occasion, proving that vegetarian cooking can be both simple and sensational.

Transform your kitchen and your life with the Vegetarian Cookbook for Beginners 2024. Whether you're looking to improve your health, simplify your meal prep, or discover new culinary delights, this cookbook is your ultimate guide to a brighter, healthier future.

The Vegetarian Cookbook for Beginners 2024 is more than just a collection of recipes; it is a comprehensive guide designed to transform your eating habits and enhance your overall well-being. This cookbook serves multiple functions: a nutritional guide, a culinary instructor, and a lifestyle enhancer. Here's a detailed analysis of its importance and why it deserves a spot in your cookbook collection.

Nutritional Benefits

Vegetarian diets are renowned for their health benefits, including reduced risk of chronic diseases such as heart disease, diabetes, and certain cancers. This cookbook meticulously curates recipes that ensure a balanced intake of essential nutrients, often overlooked in a typical vegetarian diet. It emphasizes protein-rich legumes, whole grains, and a variety of vegetables, ensuring you receive a well-rounded diet. Each recipe includes nutritional information, helping you understand the value of what you're consuming and how it contributes to your overall health.

Ease of Use

Transitioning to a vegetarian diet can be daunting, especially for beginners. The Vegetarian Cookbook for Beginners 2024 is crafted with simplicity in mind. It breaks down complex recipes into easy-to-follow steps, making it accessible even for those who are new to cooking. The book also provides tips on essential kitchen tools and pantry staples, ensuring you are well-equipped to embark on your vegetarian journey.

Variety and Flavor

One common misconception about vegetarian diets is that they are bland or monotonous. This cookbook dispels that myth by offering a wide array of recipes from different cuisines, ensuring that your meals are always exciting and full of flavor. From hearty breakfasts to sumptuous dinners and delightful desserts, this cookbook covers all meals of the day. The use of diverse spices and ingredients not only enhances the flavor but also introduces you to global culinary traditions, making your cooking experience rich and varied.

Environmental Impact

By choosing a vegetarian lifestyle, you contribute to a more sustainable planet. This cookbook subtly weaves in the importance of reducing meat consumption for environmental reasons, providing readers with an added sense of purpose. The recipes are designed to make the most of plant-based ingredients, reducing waste and encouraging sustainable eating practices.

Personal Stories and Inspiration

The Vegetarian Cookbook for Beginners 2024 is interspersed with personal stories and testimonials from individuals who have successfully transitioned to a vegetarian diet. These narratives provide inspiration and practical advice, making the cookbook more relatable and motivating. For example, a story of a busy professional who improved her health and energy levels by following the cookbook's guidance can inspire readers to make similar positive changes.

Practical Tips and Meal Planning

In addition to recipes, the cookbook offers invaluable advice on meal planning and preparation. It includes weekly meal plans, shopping lists, and batch cooking tips, making it easier to integrate vegetarian meals into your daily routine. This practical approach saves time and ensures you always have healthy, delicious meals on hand.

Making the switch to a vegetarian diet can have several advantages.

It often leads to a healthier lifestyle, with increased intake of essential vitamins, minerals, and fiber. Many studies have shown that a well-planned vegetarian diet can reduce the risk of chronic diseases such as heart disease, diabetes, and certain cancers. Additionally, reducing meat consumption is a powerful way to lessen your environmental footprint, contributing to a more sustainable plane

What to Expect

This cookbook is divided into easy-to-follow sections, each tailored to guide you through different aspects of vegetarian cooking:

Getting Started: Learn the basics of vegetarian nutrition, including essential nutrients and how to ensure you're getting a balanced diet.

Pantry Staples: A comprehensive guide to stocking your kitchen with vegetarian essentials, from grains and legumes to herbs and spices.

Breakfasts and Brunches: Kickstart your day with energizing and wholesome vegetarian breakfast options.

Lunches and Light Meals: Quick and easy recipes perfect for midday meals, whether you're at home or on the go.

Dinners: Hearty and satisfying dishes that will please even the most dedicated meat-lovers.

Snacks and Appetizers: Tasty bites and small plates for any occasion.

Desserts: Indulgent yet healthy treats to satisfy your sweet tooth.

Tips and Techniques: Practical advice on meal planning, preparation, and cooking techniques to make your vegetarian journey seamless and enjoyable.

Simple and Delicious Recipes

Each recipe in this cookbook is designed to be simple and approachable, using readily available ingredients. Whether you're a novice in the kitchen or an experienced cook looking to expand your repertoire, you'll find recipes that are easy to follow and delightfully delicious.

Embark on Your Vegetarian Journey

Embrace the vibrant and diverse world of vegetarian cuisine. With The Beginner's Vegetarian Cookbook, you'll discover that going meat-free doesn't mean sacrificing flavor or satisfaction. Instead, it's an opportunity to explore new foods, discover creative cooking techniques, and enjoy meals that are both good for you and the planet.

Happy   cooking!

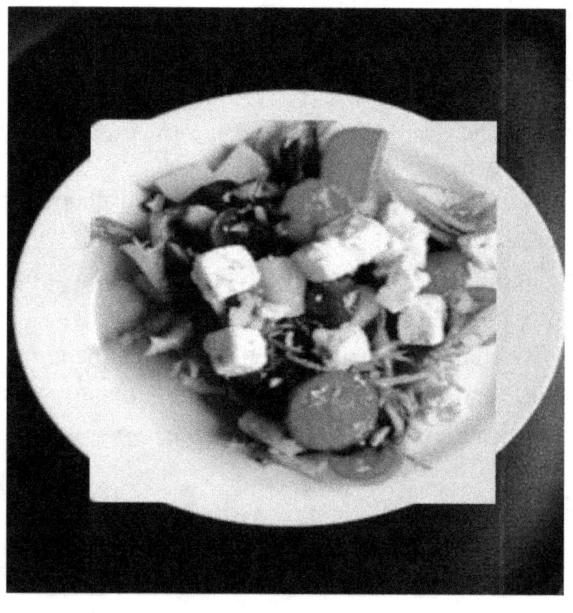

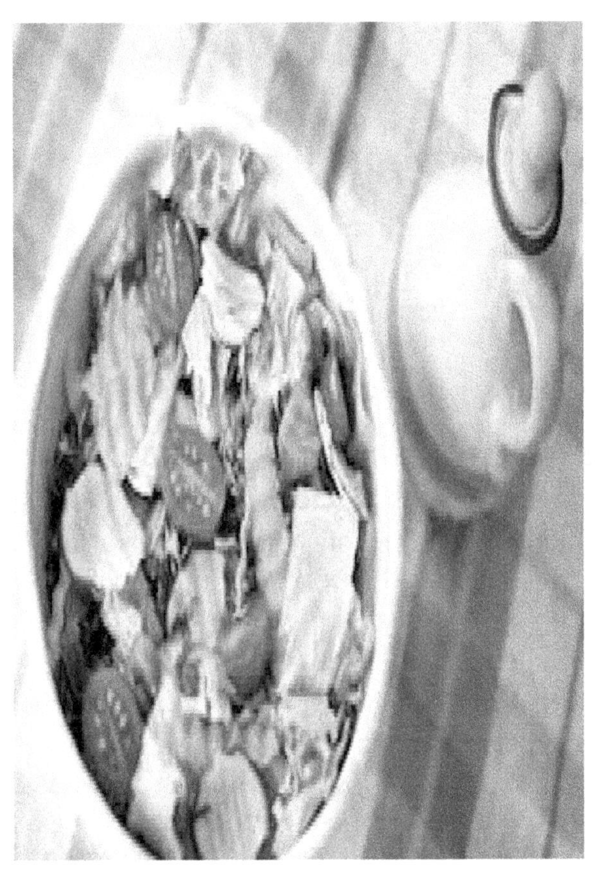

CHAPTER ONE

Benefits of vegetarianism

Adopting a vegetarian diet offers numerous benefits, encompassing health, environmental, and ethical aspects. These are few benefits to help you

Health Benefits

Nutrient-Rich Diet: Vegetarian diets tend to be high in essential nutrients such as fiber, vitamins (especially C and E), folic acid, magnesium, and phytochemicals, contributing to overall health and well-being.

Lower Risk of Chronic Diseases: A well-planned vegetarian diet is associated with a lower risk of chronic illnesses, including heart disease, hypertension, type 2 diabetes, and certain cancers

Weight Management: Vegetarians often have lower body mass indexes (BMIs) and a reduced risk of obesity. Plant-based diets are typically lower in calories and high in fiber, which promotes satiety and helps maintain a healthy weight.

Improved Digestion: High fiber intake from fruits, vegetables, and whole grains supports healthy digestion and prevents constipation.

Better Blood Sugar Control: Vegetarian diets can improve blood sugar levels and insulin sensitivity, reducing the risk of type 2 diabetes.

Cholesterol and Blood Pressure: A plant-based diet is effective in lowering LDL cholesterol (the "bad" cholesterol) and maintaining healthy blood pressure levels.

Environmental Benefits

Reduced Carbon Footprint: Plant-based diets generally have a lower carbon footprint compared to diets high in animal products. Livestock farming is a significant source of greenhouse gas emissions.

Conservation of Water: Producing plant foods requires less water than raising animals for meat. A vegetarian diet helps conserve water resources

Less Land Use: Growing plants for direct human consumption requires less land compared to growing feed for livestock, promoting more efficient use of land resources.

Lower Pollution Levels: Animal agriculture contributes to soil and water pollution through runoff of pesticides, fertilizers, and animal waste. A vegetarian diet helps reduce these environmental pollutants.

Ethical Benefit

Animal Welfare: Adopting a vegetarian diet reduces the demand for meat and, consequently, the number of animals raised and slaughtered for food. This choice supports animal welfare and humane treatment.

Sustainable Food Systems: Vegetarianism can promote more sustainable and ethical food systems by reducing the reliance on factory farming practices that are often associated with poor animal welfare and environmental degradation.

Other Benefits

Economic Savings: Plant-based foods are often less expensive than meat, allowing individuals to save money on their grocery bills.
Diverse and Flavorful Cuisine: A vegetarian diet encourages exploring a wide variety of foods, flavors, and culinary traditions, enhancing your palate and culinary skills.
By choosing a vegetarian lifestyle, you can experience these benefits while contributing positively to your health, the environment, and ethical food practices.

 A guide and tools to setting up a vegetarian kitchen
Setting up a vegetarian kitchen involves stocking up on essential ingredients, tools, and appliances to create delicious and nutritious meat-free meals. Here's a guide to help you get started

Plant-Based Staples: Fill your pantry with grains like quinoa, rice, and pasta, along with legumes such as lentils, beans, and chickpeas. They offer fiber, protein and other necessary elements

Fresh Produce: Load up on a variety of fruits and vegetables, both fresh and frozen. Opt for seasonal produce to ensure freshness and affordability.

Herbs and Spices: Enhance the flavor of your dishes with a diverse selection of herbs and spices. Essentials include garlic, onion, basil, oregano, cumin, turmeric, and paprika.

Plant-Based-Proteins: Incorporate tofu, tempeh, seitan, and plant-based meat substitutes into your meals for protein diversity. These products mimic the texture and taste of meat while being cruelty-free.

Healthy Fats: Stock up on sources of healthy fats like avocados, nuts, seeds, and olive oil. These are crucial for brain function and overall health.

Dairy Alternatives: Replace dairy products with plant-based alternatives such as almond milk, soy milk, coconut yogurt, and vegan cheese. These options provide calcium and other essential nutrients without animal-derived ingredients.

Whole Grains: For more fibre and minerals, opt for whole grains rather than processed grains, Include options like whole wheat bread, brown rice, oats, and barley in your kitchen.

Nutritional Yeast: This vegan staple adds a cheesy flavor to dishes and is a good source of vitamins, especially B12.

Kitchen Tools: Equip your kitchen with essential tools like a good knife set, cutting boards, pots, pans, blender, food processor, and vegetable spiralizer. Meal preparation will be more effective and easier with these equipment

Recipe Books and Resources: Invest in vegetarian and vegan cookbooks or explore online resources for inspiration and recipes. Experimenting with new dishes will keep your meals exciting and diverse.

By following these guidelines, you'll be well-equipped to create delicious and satisfying vegetarian meals in your kitchen.

Non-Dairy Milk Alternatives: If you enjoy milk, have a variety of non-dairy options such as almond, soy, oat, or coconut milk for cooking and baking.

Kitchen Tools: Invest in kitchen tools like a good blender, food processor, sharp knives, and quality cookware to make meal preparation easier.

Recipe Inspiration: Explore vegetarian cookbooks, websites, and apps for inspiration and new ideas. Experiment with different cuisines to keep meals exciting.

Meal Planning: Plan your meals ahead of time to ensure you have the ingredients you need and to minimize food waste.

Stay Informed: Keep educating yourself about nutrition to ensure you're meeting your dietary needs as a vegetarian. Consider consulting a dietitian if needed.

Remember to enjoy the journey of exploring new ingredients and flavors in your vegetarian kitchen

Tips to success in the kitchen

Success in the kitchen comes down to a combination of preparation, technique, and creativity. The following advice can help you succeed in the kitchen

Read the Recipe Thoroughly: Before you start cooking, read the recipe from beginning to end to familiarize yourself with the steps and ingredients.

Prep Ingredients in Advance: Chop vegetables, measure ingredients, and prepare any necessary components before you begin cooking. This will streamline the cooking process and prevent last-minute scrambling.

Keep Your Workspace Organized: Clear clutter from your workspace and keep your ingredients and tools within reach. A clean and organized kitchen will help you stay focused and efficient.

Use the Right Tools: Invest in quality kitchen tools and utensils that are suitable for the task at hand. Sharp knives, sturdy pots and pans, and reliable kitchen gadgets can make a significant difference in your cooking experience.

Master Basic Techniques: Learn fundamental cooking techniques such as chopping,sautéing, roasting, boiling, and grilling. These skills form the foundation of countless recipes and will empower you to tackle a wide range of dishes.

Season Food Properly: Taste your food as you cook and adjust seasoning accordingly. Salt enhances flavors, but be mindful not to overdo it. Experiment with herbs, spices, and other seasonings to add depth and complexity to your dishes.

Don't Be Afraid to Experiment: Cooking is a creative process, so don't hesitate to experiment with new ingredients, flavors, and cooking methods. Some of the best dishes are born from spontaneous innovation.

Practice Patience: Cooking requires patience and attention to detail. Avoid rushing through recipes and give your food the time it needs to cook properly. Practice patience, and you'll be rewarded with delicious results.
Clean as You Go: Wash dishes, wipe down countertops, and tidy up spills as you cook to maintain a clean and organized workspace. Cleaning as you go will make the post-cooking cleanup much more manageable.
Enjoy the Process: Cooking should be enjoyable and rewarding. Embrace the creative expression and sensory experience of preparing meals, and don't forget to savor the fruits of your labor with friends and family.

Setting up a vegetarian kitchen involves stocking up on essential ingredients, tools, and appliances to create delicious and nutritious meat-free meals. Here's a guide to help you get started:

Plant-Based Staples: Fill your pantry with grains like quinoa, rice, and pasta, along with legumes such as lentils, beans, and chickpeas. These provide protein, fibre, and vital nutrients.

Fresh Produce: Load up on a variety of fruits and vegetables, both fresh and frozen. Opt for seasonal produce to ensure freshness and affordability.

Herbs and Spices: Enhance the flavor of your dishes with a diverse selection of herbs and spices. Essentials include garlic, onion, basil, oregano, cumin, turmeric, and paprika.

Plant-Based Proteins: Incorporate tofu, tempeh, seitan, and plant-based meat substitutes into your meals for protein diversity. These products mimic the texture and taste of meat while being cruelty-free.

Healthy Fats: Stock up on sources of healthy fats like avocados, nuts, seeds, and olive oil. These are crucial for brain function and overall health.

CHAPTER TWO

BREAKFAST DELIGHT:

Veggie Omelet: A step-by-step guide to making a fluffy omelet packed with vegetables

Here's a step-by-step guide to making a classic veggie omelet:

Ingredients:

3 large eggs

1/4 cup diced bell peppers (any color)

1/4 cup diced onion

1/4 cup diced tomatoes

1/4 cup chopped spinach

Salt and pepper to taste

1 tablespoon olive oil Grated cheese (optional)

Instructions:

1. Prep the Vegetables: Wash and dice the bell peppers, onion, tomatoes, and spinach. Set aside.
2. Beat the Eggs: Crack the eggs into a bowl and beat them lightly with a fork or whisk until well combined. Season with salt and pepper to taste

3. Heat the Pan: Place a non-stick skillet over medium heat and add the olive oil. Allow the oil to heat up for a minute.

4. Sauté the Vegetables: Add the diced bell peppers and onion to the skillet and sauté for 2-3 minutes, or until they begin to soften. Add the diced tomatoes and chopped spinach, and continue to cook for another 1-2 minutes. Add salt and pepper to taste.

5. Pour in the Eggs: Once the vegetables are cooked, spread them evenly across the bottom of the skillet. Pour the beaten eggs over the vegetables, making sure they are evenly distributed.

6. Cook the Omelet: Let the eggs cook undisturbed for 2-3 minutes, or until the edges start to set. Using a spatula, gently lift the edges of the omelet and tilt the skillet to allow the uncooked eggs to flow to the bottom.

7. Add Cheese (Optional): If desired, sprinkle grated cheese over one half of the omelet.

8. Fold and Serve: Once the eggs are fully set but still slightly moist on top, use a spatula to fold one half of the omelet over the other, covering the cheese if added. Let the omelet cook for another 1-2 minutes, or until the cheese is melted and the eggs are cooked to your desired doneness.

9. Serve Hot: Slide the omelet onto a plate and serve immediately. Garnish with fresh herbs, if desired.

10. Enjoy your fluffy veggie omelette packed with colorful vegetables!

Overnight Oats with Fruit and Nuts: Easy, nutritious, and customizable overnight oats recipes.

Overnight oats are indeed a versatile and nutritious breakfast option! Here's a simple recipe you can try:

Ingredients

- 1/2 cup rolled oats
- 1/2 cup milk (dairy or non-dairy)
- 1/4 cup Greek yogurt (optional, for creaminess)
- 1 tablespoon of optionally sweetened maple syrup or honey
- 1/4 teaspoon vanilla extract
- A handful of mixed fruits (such as berries, sliced bananas, or diced apples)
- A handful of nuts or seeds (such as almonds, walnuts, or chia seeds)
- Pinch of cinnamon (optional)

Instructions:

1. In a jar or container, combine the rolled oats, milk, Greek yogurt, honey or maple syrup, and vanilla extract. Stir well to combine.
2. Add your choice of fruits and nuts on top of the oat mixture.
3. Sprinkle with a pinch of cinnamon, if desired.
4. Cover the jar or container and refrigerate overnight, or for at least 4 hours.
5. In the morning, give the oats a good stir and enjoy them cold or heat them up in the microwave if you prefer warm oats.
6. Feel free to customize the recipe according to your preferences by adding different fruits, nuts, seeds, or flavorings

Avocado Toast Variations: Different ways to prepare avocado toast, from simple to gourmet.

Certainly! Avocado toast is a versatile dish with endless variations. Here are some ideas:

1. Classic Avocado Toast: Mashed avocado spread on toasted bread, seasoned with salt, pepper, and a squeeze of lemon juice.

2. Egg and Avocado Toast: Top your avocado toast with a fried, poached, or scrambled egg for added protein and flavor.

3. Tomato and Avocado Toast: Add slices of fresh tomato on top of the mashed avocado for a burst of juiciness and color.

4. Smoked Salmon Avocado Toast: Layer smoked salmon over the mashed avocado and top with capers and red onion for a luxurious twist.

5. Avocado and Bacon Toast: Crisp up some bacon and place it on top of the mashed avocado for a savory and indulgent treat.

6. Avocado and Feta Toast: Sprinkle crumbled feta cheese over the mashed avocado and finish with a drizzle of balsamic glaze for a tangy kick.

7. Mushroom and Avocado Toast: Sautéed mushrooms make a delicious topping for avocado toast, especially when seasoned with garlic and thyme.

8. Avocado and Radish Toast: Thinly slice radishes and arrange them over the mashed avocado for a crunchy texture and peppery flavor.

9. Avocado and Pesto Toast: Spread pesto over the mashed avocado for a burst of herbaceous flavor, and top with cherry tomatoes or pine nuts for extra crunch.

10. Avocado and Sriracha Toast: Drizzle sriracha sauce over the mashed avocado for a spicy kick, and garnish with cilantro and sesame seeds.

11. Avocado and Goat Cheese Toast: Spread creamy goat cheese over the mashed

avocado and sprinkle with chopped herbs like basil or chives.

12. Avocado and Shrimp Toast: Top your avocado toast with cooked shrimp and a squeeze of lime juice for a refreshing and light

13. Vegetable Frittata Recipe A vegetable frittata is a versatile and hearty dish that's perfect for any breakfast table. It's simple to prepare and can be tailored to include your preferred veggies.

Ingredients:

- 8 large eggs
- 1/2 cup milk (whole, 2%, or plant-based)
- 1 cup bell peppers, diced (red, green, or yellow)
- 1 cup zucchini, diced
- 1 cup spinach, chopped
- 1/2 cup onion, finely chopped
- 2 cloves garlic, minced
- 1/2 cup cherry tomatoes, halved
- 1/2 cup shredded cheese (cheddar, mozzarella, or feta)
- 2 tablespoons olive oil
- Salt and pepper to taste
- Fresh herbs (optional: parsley, basil, or chives)

Instructions:

1. Preheat Oven: Preheat your oven to 375°F (190°C).
2. Prepare Vegetables: In a large skillet, warm the olive oil over medium heat. Add the onions and garlic, cooking until softened, about 2-3 minutes.
   - Add bell peppers, zucchini, and cook for another 5 minutes until they start to soften.
   - Stir in spinach and cherry tomatoes, cooking until the spinach wilts. Season with salt and pepper to taste. Remove from heat.
3. Prepare Egg Mixture:
   - Whisk the eggs and milk together thoroughly in a sizable bowl.
   - Stir in the shredded cheese and fresh herbs if using. Add a dash of pepper and salt for seasoning
4. Combine and Cook:
   - Add the cooked vegetables to the egg mixture and stir to combine.
   - Spoon the batter onto a baking dish or skillet that is safe to use in the oven.
5. Bake:

- Bake for 20 to 25 minutes, or until the frittata is set and has a golden brown top, in a preheated oven.
- To ensure doneness, test the middle with a toothpick or knife; it should come out clean.
- Serve:Before slicing, let the frittata cool for a few minutes.

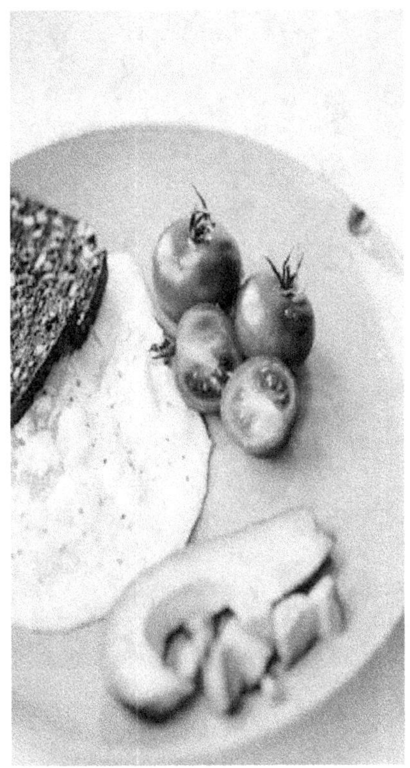

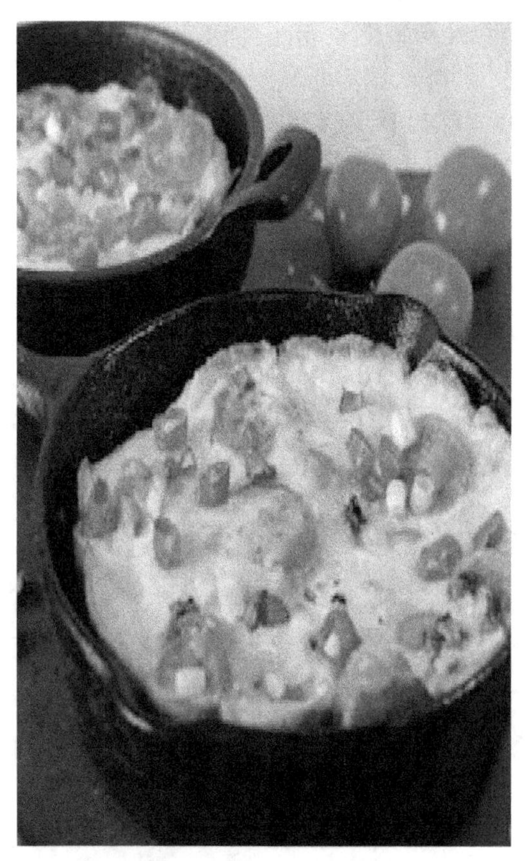

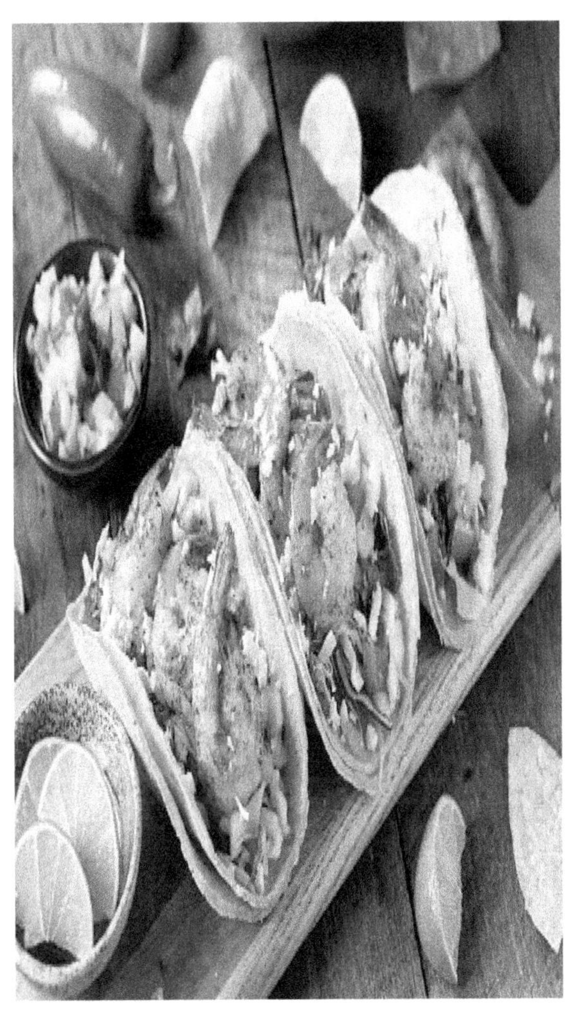

CHAPTER THREE

APPETIZERS AND SNACKS.

Spinach and Feta Stuffed Mushrooms: Savory mushrooms filled with a delicious spinach and feta mixture.Here's a simple and delicious recipe for Spinach and Feta Stuffed Mushrooms:

Ingredients:

- 20 large mushrooms (such as white button or cremini), stems removed and finely chopped
- 1 tablespoon olive oil
- 1 small onion, finely chopped
- 2 cloves garlic, minced
- 4 cups fresh spinach, chopped
- 1/2 cup feta cheese, crumbled
- 1/4 cup breadcrumbs
- 1/4 teaspoon salt
- 1/4 teaspoon black pepper
- 1/4 teaspoon dried oregano
- 1/4 teaspoon dried thyme
- 2 tablespoons grated Parmesan cheese (optional)

Instructions:

1. Preheat the Oven: Preheat your oven to 375°F (190°C). A baking sheet can be lightly greased or lined with parchment paper.

2. Prepare the Mushrooms: Clean the mushroom caps with a damp paper towel to remove any dirt. Remove the stems with care, then cut them finely.

3. Cook the Filling:
   - In a large skillet, warm the olive oil over medium heat.
   - Add the chopped mushroom stems and onion. Sauté for about 5 minutes, or until the onion becomes translucent.
   - Incorporate the garlic and cook for a further minute.
   - Add the chopped spinach and simmer for two to three minutes, or until it wilts.
   - After taking the skillet from the burner, let the mixture to cool somewhat.

4. Mix the Filling: In a medium bowl, combine the cooked spinach mixture with the feta cheese, breadcrumbs, salt, black pepper, oregano, and thyme. Mix until well combined.

5. Stuff the Mushrooms: Spoon the spinach and feta mixture into the mushroom caps, pressing down lightly to fill each cap generously.

6. Bake the Mushrooms: Arrange the stuffed mushrooms on the prepared baking sheet. Sprinkle the tops with grated Parmesan cheese if using. Bake for 20 to 25 minutes, or until the filling is golden brown and the mushrooms are soft, in a preheated oven.

7. To serve, take out of the oven and allow to cool a little. Enjoy these savory stuffed mushrooms as an appetizer or a side dish!

8. Enjoy your Spinach and Feta Stuffed Mushrooms!

Homemade Hummus with Veggie Sticks: A classic hummus recipe paired with fresh vegetable sticksTips:

Here are some tips for making homemade hummus and pairing it with fresh vegetable sticks:

Classic Hummus Recipe:

Ingredients:

- 1 can (15 oz) rinsed and drained chickpeas (garbanzo beans)
- 1/4 cup fresh lemon juice (about 1 large lemon)
- 1/4 cup well-stirred tahini
- 1 small garlic clove, minced
- 2 tablespoons of extra virgin olive oil, plus additional to dress.
- 1/2 teaspoon ground cumin
- Salt to taste
- 2-3 tablespoons water
- Paprika, for garnish (optional)

Instructions:

1. Blend Ingredients: In a food processor, combine tahini and lemon juice. After one minute, scrape down the edges and continue processing for thirty seconds.
2. Add Ingredients: Add the olive oil, minced garlic, cumin, and a pinch of salt to the whipped tahini and lemon juice. Process for 30 seconds, scrape the sides, and process for another 30 seconds or until well-blended.
3. Chickpeas: Add half of the chickpeas to the food processor and process for 1 minute. Scrape sides and bottom of the bowl, then add the remaining chickpeas and process until thick and smooth (1-2 minutes).
4. Adjust Consistency: With the food processor running, add 2-3 tablespoons of water until you reach the desired consistency.
5. Season: Taste and adjust with more salt, lemon juice, or olive oil as needed.
6. Serve: Transfer to a serving bowl, drizzle with a bit of olive oil, and sprinkle with paprika if desire
7. Tips for Pairing with Vegetable Sticks:
1. Veggie Variety: Use a variety of vegetables for a colorful and nutritious platter. Good options include carrots, celery, cucumber, bell peppers, cherry tomatoes, and radishes.

2. Prep Ahead: Wash and cut your vegetables ahead of time to make serving easy. Store them in cold water in the fridge to keep them crisp.

3. Uniform Size: Cut vegetable sticks into uniform sizes for easy dipping.

4. Presentation: Arrange the vegetable sticks around the hummus bowl in a visually appealing way. Use a large platter or a wooden board for a rustic look.

5. Additional Toppings: Enhance the hummus with additional toppings like whole chickpeas, a drizzle of extra virgin olive oil, a sprinkle of paprika, or chopped fresh herbs like parsley or cilantro.

6. Enjoy your homemade hummus with fresh vegetable sticks for a healthy and delicious snack!

Here's a recipe for making fresh and zesty guacamole and salsa, along with homemade baked tortilla chips:

Guacamole and Salsa with Baked Tortilla Chips: Fresh and zesty guacamole and salsa served with homemade baked tortilla chips

Guacamole Recipe:

Ingredients:

- 3 ripe avocados
- 1 small onion, finely chopped
- 1-2 tomatoes, diced
- Minced one or two jalapeños (seed removed for reduced heat)
- 2-3 tablespoons fresh cilantro, chopped
- Juice of 1 lime
- Salt to taste

Instructions:

Prepare Avocados: Cut the avocados in half, remove the pits, and scoop the flesh into a mixing bowl.

- Mash Avocados: Mash the avocados with a fork to your desired consistency (chunky or smooth).
- Mix Ingredients: Add the chopped onion, tomatoes, jalapeños, cilantro, and lime juice to the mashed avocados.
- Season: Add salt to taste and mix everything together until well combined.
- Serve: Transfer to a serving bowl. Garnish with additional cilantro or a sprinkle of chili

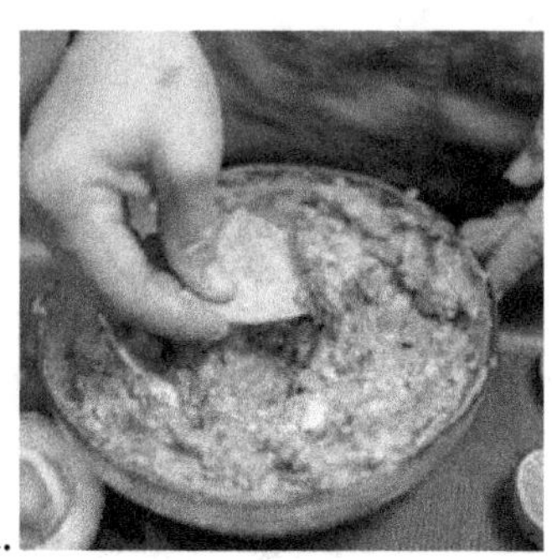

powder if desired.

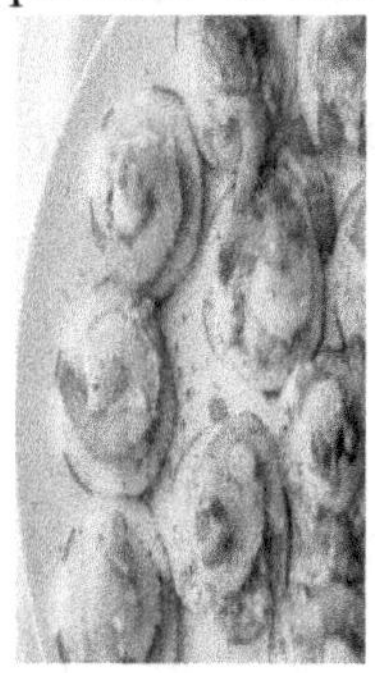

Salsa Recipe:

Ingredients:

- 4-5 ripe tomatoes, finely diced
- 1 small onion, finely chopped
- Mince 1-2 jalapeños, removing seeds for less heat.
- 2-3 tablespoons fresh cilantro, chopped
- Juice of 1 lime
- Salt to taste
- Optional: 1-2 cloves garlic, minced

Instructions:

- Combine Ingredients: In a mixing bowl, combine the diced tomatoes, chopped onion, minced jalapeños, cilantro, and lime juice.
- Season: Add salt to taste and mix well.
- Optional Garlic: If using, add the minced garlic and mix until well combined.
- Chill: To let the flavors melt together, place in the refrigerator for at least half an hour.
- Serve: Transfer to a serving bowl. Garnish with additional cilantro if desired.

Baked Tortilla Chips

Here's a recipe for making Caprese Skewers with a balsamic glaze, which makes for a simple and elegant appetizer:

Ingredients:

- 1 pint cherry tomatoes
- 1 pound fresh mozzarella balls (bocconcini or ciliegine)
- Fresh basil leaves
- Balsamic glaze (store-bought or homemade)
- Wooden or metal skewers
- Instructions:
- Prep Ingredients: Rinse the cherry tomatoes and fresh basil leaves. Drain the mozzarella balls if they are in liquid.

- Assemble Skewers: Thread one cherry tomato, one mozzarella ball, and one basil leaf onto each skewer. Repeat this pattern until the skewer is filled, leaving some space at the end for handling.
- Tip: If using long skewers, you can repeat the pattern multiple times per skewer.
- Arrange on Platter: Place the assembled skewers on a serving platter in a visually appealing manner.
- Drizzle with Balsamic Glaze: Just before serving, drizzle the skewers with balsamic glaze. Be careful not to overdo it, as the glaze can be quite flavorful.
- Serve Immediately: These are best served fresh. If you need to prepare them a little in advance, store them in the fridge and drizzle with the glaze just before serving.

Balsamic Glaze(Optional Homemade Version):

Ingredients:

- 1 cup balsamic vinegar
- 2 tablespoons honey or brown sugar

Instructions:

Combine Ingredients: In a small saucepan, combine the balsamic vinegar and honey (or brown sugar).
Simmer: Bring to a gentle boil over medium heat, then reduce the heat to low and let it simmer.

Reduce: Stir occasionally and simmer until the vinegar has reduced by about half and has a syrupy consistency (this usually takes 10-15 minutes).
Cool: Let the glaze cool slightly before drizzling over the skewers. The more it cools, the thicker it gets.
Enjoy your Caprese Skewers with Balsamic Glaze, a perfect blend of fresh flavors and elegant balsamic glaze

CHAPTER FOUR

Wholesome Salads

Quinoa and Roasted Vegetable Salad: A protein-packed salad with roasted vegetables and quinoa.

Here's a recipe for a wholesome Quinoa and Roasted Vegetable Salad that's both protein-packed and full of flavor:

Ingredients:

For the Salad:

1 cup quinoa, rinsed

2 cups water or vegetable broth

1 red bell pepper, chopped

1 yellow bell pepper, chopped

1 zucchini, chopped

1 red onion, chopped

1 cup cherry tomatoes, halved

1 cup broccoli florets

2 tablespoons olive oil

Salt and pepper to taste

1/4 cup chopped fresh parsley (optional)

1/4 cup crumbled feta cheese (optional)

For the Dressing:

1/4 cup olive oil

2 tablespoons balsamic vinegar

1 tablespoon lemon juice

1 garlic clove, minced

1 teaspoon Dijon mustard

Salt and pepper to taste

Instructions:

- Cook Quinoa:
- Rinse the quinoa and put it in a medium pot with some water or vegetable broth.
- After bringing to a boil, lower the heat to a simmer, cover, and let the quinoa cook for approximately 15 minutes, or until the liquid has been absorbed.

- Take it off the heat and leave it covered for five minutes. Using a fork, fluff and allow to cool.
- Roast Vegetables:
- Preheat your oven to 425°F (220°C).
- Place the chopped bell peppers, zucchini, red onion, cherry tomatoes, and broccoli florets on a large baking sheet.
- Add a drizzle of two tablespoons olive oil and season with pepper and salt.
- Toss to coat the vegetables evenly.
- Roast in the preheated oven for about 20-25 minutes, or until the vegetables are tender and slightly charred, stirring halfway through.
- Prepare Dressing:
- In a small bowl, whisk together the olive oil, balsamic vinegar, lemon juice, minced garlic, Dijon mustard, salt, and pepper until well combined.
- Assemble Salad:
- In a large mixing bowl, combine the cooked quinoa and roasted vegetables.
- Toss to combine the Nosalad with the dressing after adding it.
- If desired, add the chopped fresh parsley and crumbled feta cheese.
- Serve:
- Transfer to individual plates or a serving bowl.
- You can serve this salad cold or hot.

Enjoy your Quinoa and Roasted Vegetable Salad, a nutritious and delicious meal that's perfect for any occasion

Greek Salad with Tofu Feta: A vegetarian twist on the classic Greek salad with homemade tofu feta

Ingredients:

For the Salad:

- 2 cups cherry tomatoes, halved
- 1 large cucumber, diced
- 1 green bell pepper, chopped
- 1 red bell pepper, chopped
- 1 small red onion, thinly sliced
- 1/2 cup Kalamata olives, pitted
- 1/4 cup fresh parsley, chopped veggies

For the Tofu Feta:

- 1 block firm tofu, pressed and cubed
- 1/4 cup lemon juice
- 1/4 cup apple cider vinegar
- 1/4 cup olive oil
- 1/4 cup nutritional yeast
- 1 tbsp dried oregano
- 1 tsp salt
- 1 tsp garlic powder

For the Dressing:

- 1/4 cup extra virgin olive oil
- 2 tbsp red wine vinegar
- 1 tsp dried oregano

- Salt and pepper to taste

Instructions:

Prepare the Tofu Feta:

- Press the tofu to remove excess water. Once pressed, cut it into small cubes.
- In a bowl, whisk together the lemon juice, apple cider vinegar, olive oil, nutritional yeast, oregano, salt, and garlic powder.
- Add the cubed tofu to the marinade, ensuring all pieces are well-coated. Allow it to marinade in the fridge for at least an hour, or overnight for optimal taste.

Assemble the Salad:

In a large salad bowl, combine the cherry tomatoes, cucumber, green bell pepper, red bell pepper, red onion, Kalamata olives, and parsley.

Prepare the Dressing:

- In a small mixing bowl, combine the olive oil, red wine vinegar, oregano, salt, and pepper.
- Combine Everything:
- Toss with the marinated tofu feta.

- Toss the salad lightly to combine it with the dressing after adding it.
- Serve:
- Serve immediately or let it chill in the refrigerator for about 30 minutes to allow the flavors to meld together.
- Enjoy your delicious and refreshing Greek Salad with Tofu Feta!
- Chickpea and Avocado Salad: A creamy and filling salad with chickpeas and avocado

Ingredients:

- 1 can chickpeas, drained and rinsed
- 1 ripe avocado, diced
- 1 small red onion, finely chopped
- 1 cup cherry tomatoes, halved
- 1 cucumber, diced
- 1/4 cup fresh cilantro or parsley, chopped
- Juice of 1 lime
- 2 tablespoons olive oil
- Salt and pepper to taste

Instructions:

- In a large bowl, combine the chickpeas, avocado, red onion, cherry tomatoes, cucumber, and cilantro or Mix the lime juice, olive oil, salt, and pepper in a small bowl.
- Toss the salad lightly to combine it with the dressing after adding it.

- Adjust seasoning to taste and serve immediately.
- Enjoy your creamy and filling Chickpea and Avocado Salad!
- Asian-Inspired Noodle Salad: A light and refreshing salad with noodles and an Asian-inspired dressing. Asian-Inspired Noodle Salad

Ingredients:

- 8 oz rice noodles or thin spaghetti
- 1 cup shredded carrots
- 1 cup thinly sliced red bell pepper
- 1 cup thinly sliced cucumber
- 1/2 cup chopped green onions
- 1/4 cup chopped fresh cilantro
- 1/4 cup chopped fresh mint (optional)
- 1/4 cup chopped peanuts or cashews (for garnish)
- Dressing:
- 1/4 cup soy sauce
- 2 tablespoons rice vinegar
- 1 tablespoon sesame oil
- 1 tablespoon honey or maple syrup
- 1 tablespoon lime juice
- 1 teaspoon grated fresh ginger
- 1 garlic clove, minced
- 1/2 teaspoon red pepper flakes (optional)

Instructions:

- Cook the noodles according to package instructions. To halt cooking, drain and rinse with cold water. Set aside.
- In a large bowl, combine the cooked noodles, shredded carrots, red bell pepper, cucumber, green onions, cilantro, and mint (if using).
- In a small bowl, whisk together the soy sauce, rice vinegar, sesame oil, honey or maple syrup, lime juice, ginger, garlic, and red pepper flakes.
- Pour the dressing over the noodle mixture and toss to coat evenly.
- Before serving, garnish with chopped cashews or peanuts.
- Serve immediately for a light and refreshing meal. Enjoy
-

CHAPTER FIVE

Hearty Soups and stews

Lentil Soup with Warm Spices

Ingredients :

- 1 mug dried lentils,
- irrigated onion,
- finely diced cloves garlic,
- diced carrots,
- minced celery stalks
- minced tsp ground cumin
- 1 tsp ground coriander
- 1 tsp ground turmeric
- 1 tsp ground cinnamon
- 1 tsp ground nutmeg
- 6 mugs vegetable broth
- 1 can(14.5 oz) minced tomatoes swab and pepper to taste
- 2 tbsp olive oil
- Fresh cilantro or parsley for trim(voluntary)

Instructions:

- In a large pot, warm the olive oil over medium heat. Add the celery, carrots, onion, and garlic.
- Sauté for 5 to 7 minutes or until tender.
- Stir in cumin, coriander, turmeric, cinnamon, and nutmeg.
- Cook for another nanosecond until ambrosial.
- Add lentils, vegetable broth, and minced tomatoes. Bring to a pustule.
- Reduce heat and poach,
- covered, for 30 to 35 minutes, or until the lentils are soft.
- Season with swab and pepper to taste.
- Garnish with fresh parsley or cilantro before serving, if asked .

Creamy Tomato Basil Soup

Ingredients:

- 2 tbsp olive oil
- 1 onion, diced cloves garlic,
- diced barrels(28 oz each)
- whole tomatoes with peels
- 1 mug heavy cream
- 1 mug vegetable broth mug

- finely diced fresh basil leaves swab and pepper to taste

Instructions:

- In a large pot, warm the olive oil over medium heat. Add the onion and garlic.
- Sauté for about 5 minutes, or until the onion becomes transparent.
- Add the tomatoes and their juice, along with the vegetable broth.
- Bring to a pustule, also reduce heat and poach for 20 minutes
- Using an absorption blender, purée the haze until smooth, or transfer to a blender in batches and purée until smooth.
- Return the haze to the pot.
- Stir in heavy cream and basil.
- Heat through, but don't boil.
- Season with swab and pepper to taste.
- Serve hot.

Vegetable Minestrone Ingredients

- 2 tbsp olive oil
- 1 onion, diced cloves garlic
- ,diced carrots,
- minced celery stalks
- minced zucchini
- minced potato, hulled and minced can(14.5 oz) minced tomatoes 6 mugs vegetable broth

- 1 can(15 oz) order sap, irrigated and drained mug small pasta(e.g., ditalini)
- 1tsp dried oregano
- 1 tsp dried basil swab and pepper to taste lately grated Parmesan for serving(voluntary)

Instructions :

- In a large saucepan, toast the olive oil over medium heat.
- Add the celery, carrots, onion, and garlic.
- Sauté for 5 to 7 minutes or until tender.
- Add the minced tomatoes, potato, zucchini, oregano, and basil.
- Stir and bring to a pustule.
- Reduce heat and poach, covered, for 20 minutes
- Add order sap and pasta.
- Continue to poach for another 10- 12 minutes or until pasta is tender.
- Season with swab and pepper to taste.
- Serve with grated Parmesan rubbish, if asked .

Butternut Squash and Coconut Curry Soup

Ingredients :

- 2 tbsp olive oil
- 1 onion, diced cloves garlic
- diced tbsp fresh gusto
- diced tbsp curry greasepaint
- 1 butternut squash, hulled, planted, and cubed mugs vegetable broth
- 1 can(14 oz) coconut milk swab and pepper to taste Fresh cilantro for trim(voluntary)

Instructions :

- Heat the olive oil in a big saucepan over a moderate flame.
- Add onion, garlic, and ginger.
- Boil until the onion is clear, roughly 5 minutes. After adding the curry powder, simmer for an additional minute
- .Boil for about 5 minutes, or until onion is opaque.
- Simmer onion for 5 minutes or until it becomes transparent.
- Add butternut squash and vegetable broth. Bring to a boil, then reduce heat and simmer until squash is tender, about 20-25 minutes.

- Blend the soup with a handheld blender until it's smooth.
- Alternatively, transfer the soup in batches to a blender and puree until smooth.
- Return the soup to the pot. Stir in coconut milk and heat through, but do not boil.
- Season with salt and pepper to taste.
- Garnish with fresh cilantro before serving, if desired

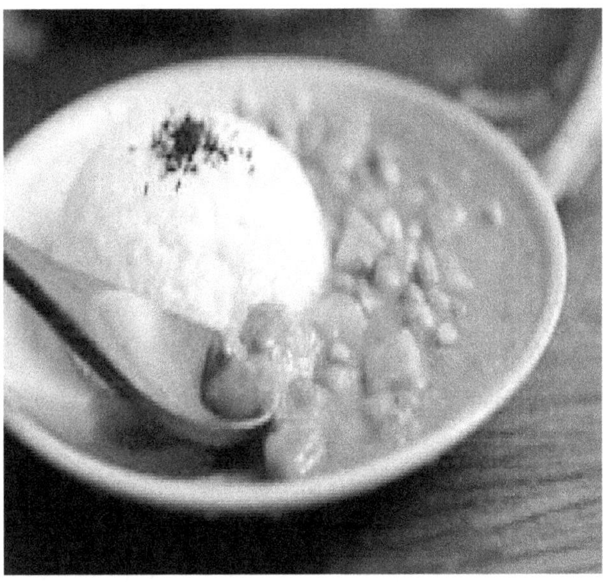

CHAPTER SIX

NOURISHING MAIN DISHES

Vegetarian Chili with Beans and Corn!

Ingredients

- 1 tablespoon olive oil
- 1 onion, chopped
- 2 cloves garlic, minced
- 1 chili pepper, chopped
- 1 can (14.5 oz) diced tomatoes
- 1 can (15 oz) of flushed and dried kidney beans is required.
- 1 can (15 oz) of cleaned and depleted dark beans
- 1 can (15 oz) corn, drained
- 2 tablespoons chili powder
- 1 teaspoon cumin
- 1 teaspoon paprika
- Salt and pepper to taste

Instructions:

- Heat olive oil in a expansive pot over medium warm. Include onion and garlic, and sauté until softened.
- Add chime pepper and cook for another 3-4 minutes.
- Stir in diced tomatoes, kidney beans, dark beans, and corn.
- Add chili powder, cumin, paprika, salt, and pepper. Mix well.
- Bring the blend to a bubble, at that point decrease warm and let it stew for 20-30 minutes.
- Adjust flavoring if required and serve hot.

Eggplant Parmesan with Marinara Sauce: is a classic Italian dish that's both comforting and tasty. Here's a basic formula for you

Ingredients:

- 1 huge eggplant, cut into 1/2-inch circular 1 glass breadcrumbs
- 1/2 glass ground Parmesan cheese

- 2 eggs, beaten
- 2 mugs marinara sauce
- 1 glass destroyed mozzarella cheese
- Fresh basil clears out for decorate (optional)

Instructions:

- Preheat your broiler to 375°F (190°C).
- Apply a cooking oil or olive oil to a preparing surface to oil it
- After putting the eggplant cuts in a strainer, salt them.
- Provide them a great roughly fifteen to twenty minutes to sit in arrange to let out additional dampness.
- Set up the breading gear in the intervals. Combine the pieces of bread and ground Parmesan cheese together in a shallow dish. Beat two eggs in a distinctive little dish.
- After giving the eggplant cuts a brief wash in cold water, wipe dry with paper towels to dry.
- Dip each eggplant cut into the beaten eggs, at that point coat it with the breadcrumb blend, squeezing delicately to adhere.
- Place the breaded eggplant cuts on the arranged heating sheet in a single layer.

- Bake the eggplant cuts in the preheated stove for 20-25 minutes, or until they are brilliant brown and tender.
- Remove the heating sheet from the broiler. Spoon marinara sauce over each eggplant cut and sprinkle destroyed mozzarella cheese on top
- Put the heating plate back in the warmed broiler and proceed preparing for ten to fifteen more a few minutes, or until the dairy item begins to bubble and liquefied.
- If wanted, beautify with new basil takes off in no time some time recently serving.
- Enjoy your custom made Eggplant Parmesan with Marinara Sauce! It sets brilliantly with a side of pasta or a green salad.

Tofu Stir-Fry with Blended: Vegetables is an incredible dish that's both sound and flavorful. Here's a basic formula for you to try:

Ingredients:

- 1 piece (14 oz) firm tofu, squeezed and cubed
- 2 tablespoons soy sauce
- 1 tablespoon sesame oil
- 2 cloves garlic, minced

- 1 teaspoon ginger, minced
- 1 chime pepper, sliced
- 1 carrot, julienned
- 1 glass broccoli florets
- 1 glass cut mushrooms
- 1 glass snow peas, trimmed
- 2 green onions, chopped (optional)
- Cooked rice or noodles, for serving

Instructions:

- Whisk the oil from sesame and soy sauce together in a little bowl.
- Put aside a huge pot or skillet ought to be warmed to medium-high warm.
- Include the chopped tofu and warm for 5 to 7 minutes, or until brilliant brown on all sides. After removing the tofu from the skillet, set it aside.
- If required, include a small additional oil to that same skillet.
- Include the ginger and garlic, minced, and mix until fragrant, almost 30 seconds.
- Add the cut chime pepper, julienned carrot, broccoli florets, cut mushrooms, and snow peas to the skillet. Stir-fry the vegetables approximately 5-7 minutes, or until they are tender and crispy.

- Return the cooked tofu to the skillet.
- Pour the soy sauce and sesame oil blend over the tofu and vegetables.
- Mix to coat everything evenly.
- Cook for an extra 2-3 minutes, permitting the flavors to merge together.
- If utilizing, sprinkle chopped green onions on beat for garnish.
- Serve the tofu stir-fry hot over cooked rice or noodles.
- Enjoy your scrumptious and nutritious Tofu Stir-Fry with Blended Vegetables! You are welcome to alter the vegetables to suit your tastes.

Mushroom risotto with Parmesan cheese :is a classic consolation dish, culminating for reveling in wealthy flavors and velvety surfaces: The grittiness of the mushrooms complements the nuttiness of the Parmesan cheese, making a delightful agreement of flavors. Would you likeTo make mushroom risotto with Parmesan cheese, you'll need

Ingredients:

- 1 container Arborio rice

- 4 glasses chicken or vegetable broth
- 2 tablespoons olive oil
- 1 onion, finely chopped
- 2 cloves garlic, minced
- 8 ounces of mushrooms (such as cremini or shiitake), sliced
- 1/2 glass dry white wine
- 1/2 container ground Parmesan cheese
- Salt and pepper to taste
- Fresh parsley, chopped (for garnish)

Instructions:

- In a pan, warm the broth over medium warm until warm.
- Keep it stewing whereas you get ready the risotto.
- In a isolated huge skillet or pot, warm the olive oil over medium warm.
- Include the chopped onion and cook until mellowed, almost 3-4 minutes
- . Include the minced garlic and cook for another minute.
- Add the cut mushrooms to the skillet and cook until they are browned and delicate, almost 5-7 minutes.
- Stir in the Arborio rice and cook for 1-2 minutes, until the rice is coated with oil and marginally translucent.

- While including the white wine, mix the rice until it is completely ingested.
- With consistent spinning begin including the warmed stock one ladleful at a time.
- Some time recently including extra sauce, let the rice splash the past addition.
- Allow each expansion of broth to be ingested by the rice some time recently including more. Proceed this prepare until the rice is rich and delicate, which ought to take approximately 20-25 minutes.
- Once the risotto is cooked to your wanted consistency, mix in the ground Parmesan cheese until softened and rich.
- For a good taste, add salt and pepper for seasoning.
- Serve the mushroom risotto hot, embellished with chopped new parsley and extra ground Parmesan cheese if
- desired.
- Enjoy your rich mushroom risotto with Parmesan cheese!

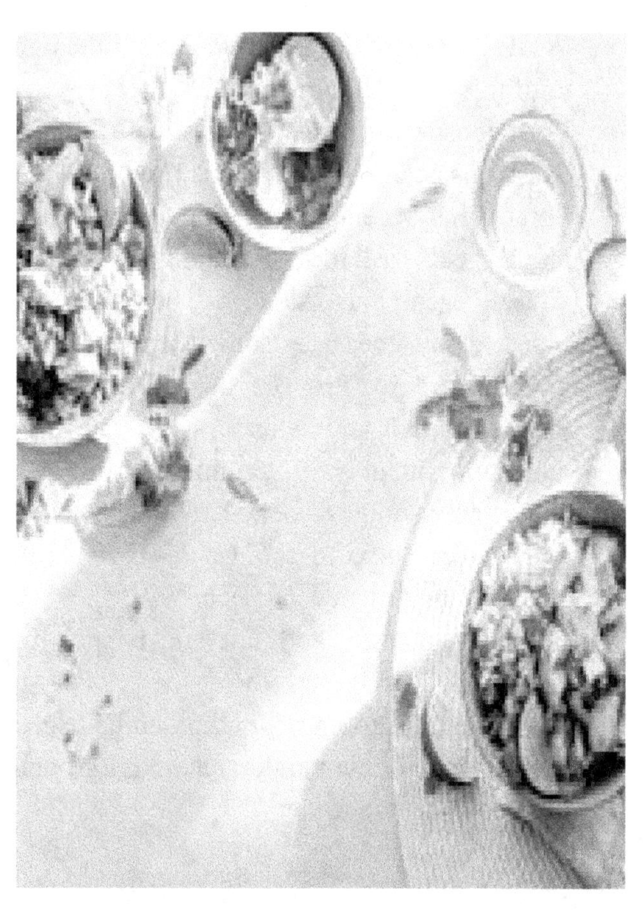

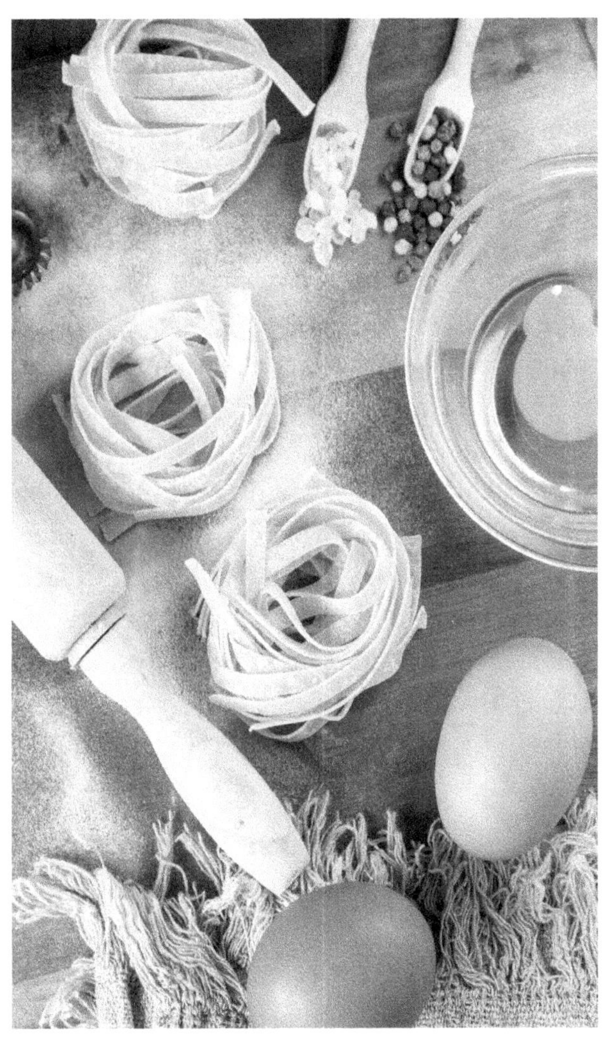

CHAPTER SEVEN

Spaghetti Aglio e Olio with Cherry Tomatoes

Spaghetti Aglio e Olio with Cherry Tomatoes. A simple yet scrumptious pasta dish with garlic, oil , and cherry tomatoes. Spaghetti Aglio e Olio with Cherry Tomatoes is a cherished Italian dish known for its simplicity and vibrant flavors. With just a sprinkle of it like garlic, olive oil, and juicy cherry tomatoes, it's easy to whip up yet incredibly satisfying.   The garlic- invested olive oil, fleeces the pasta beautifully, while the burst of agreeableness from the cherry tomatoes adds a stimulating touch. It's a classic form that will not disappoint.

Vegetable Pad Thai with Tofu A submissive interpretation of the popular

Thai pate dish with tofu and vegetables. Vegetable Pad Thai with Tofu This dish offers a pleasurable mix of flavors with the agreeableness of tamarind sauce, the tanginess of lime, and the crunchiness of peanuts. Tofu adds a protein boost, while the variety of vegetables provides both texture and nutrition. If you need a form or any tips on making it,,

Then, here is a introductory form of preparing Vegetable Pad Thai with Tofu

Ingredients:

- 200g rice polls
- 200g establishment tofu, pressed and cubed soupspoons
- vegetable oil
- 2 cloves garlic, diced small onion, thinly sliced red bell pepper, thinly sliced carrot, julienned mugs bean sprouts
- 3 green onions, diced
- 4 mug diced peanuts Lime wedges, for serving For the sauce
- 3 soupspoons soy sauce
- 2 soupspoons tamarind paste
- 2 soupspoons brown sugar
- 1 teaspoon rice ginger
- 1 tablespoon sriracha(voluntary, for heat)

Instructions :

- Cook the rice polls according to package instructions.
- Drain and set away.
- In a small coliseum, mix together the ingredients for the sauce: soy sauce,

tamarind paste, brown sugar, rice ginger, and sriracha. Set away.

- Heat 1 teaspoon of oil in a large visage or wok over medium-high heat.
- Add the tofu cells and cook until golden brown on all sides.
- Remove tofu from the visage and set away.
- In the same visage, add another teaspoon of oil
- Add the diced garlic and sliced onion, and cook until softened.
- Add the sliced bell pepper and julienned carrot to the visage, and stir- shindig for a many twinkles until slightly softened.
- Add the cooked rice polls and tofu back to the visage, along with the bean sprouts and diced green onions.
- Pour the sauce over the polls and tofu, and toss everything together until well concerted and hotted
- Serve the Vegetable Pad Thai briskly, garnished with diced peanuts and lime wedges on the side.
- Enjoy your succulent Vegetable Pad Thai with Tofu! Let me know if you have any questions or need further backing.

One- Pot Creamy Mushroom Pasta : A hassle-free pasta dish cooked in one pot with mushrooms and a delicate sauce. Then, here is a simple form :

Ingredients:

- 8 oz(225g) pasta(similar as spaghetti or fettuccine)
- 2 soupspoons olive oil
- 8 oz(225g) mushrooms, sliced(use your favorite variety) cloves garlic, diced mugs vegetable broth
- 1 mug heavy cream mug grated Parmesan rubbish swab and pepper to taste Fresh parsley, diced(voluntary, for trim)

Instructions:

- In a large pot or deep skillet, toast the olive oil over medium heat.
- Add the sliced mushrooms and diced garlic, and sauté until the mushrooms are golden brown and tender.
- Add the pasta to the pot, followed by the vegetable broth and heavy cream.
- Stir to combine.
- Bring the admixture to a pustule, also reduce the heat to medium-low and let it poach uncovered, stirring sometimes, until the pasta is cooked and the sauce has

thickened, about 10- 12 twinkles. Once the pasta is cooked to your relish and the sauce has thickened, stir in the grated Parmesan rubbish until melted and delicate.

- Season with swab and pepper to taste.
- Remove the pot from the heat and let it sit for a many hours to allow the sauce to cake further.
- Serve the One- Pot Creamy Mushroom Pasta briskly, garnished with diced fresh parsley if asked . Enjoy your hassle-free and succulent delicate mushroom pasta! Let me know if you have any questions or need farther backing.

Mexican- Inspired Quinoa Bowl : A vibrant and nutritional quinoa coliseum with Mexican- inspired flavors. Then is a form for a Mexican- Inspired Quinoa Bowl

Ingredients :

- 1 mug quinoa, irrigated mugs vegetable broth or water
- 1 teaspoon olive oil.
- 1 onion, minced cloves garlic, diced red bell pepper,
- minced mug sludge kernels(fresh, frozen, or canned)
- can(15 oz) black sap, drained and irrigated tablespoon ground cumin

- 1 tablespoon chili greasepaint swab and pepper to taste
- Juice of 1 lime Fresh cilantro, diced, for garnish Avocado slices, for garnish Salsa, for serving voluntary condiments minced tomatoes, sliced jalapeños, tattered rubbish, sour cream

Instructions :

- In a medium saucepan, combine the irrigated quinoa and vegetable broth or water.
- Bring to a pustule, also reduce the heat to low, cover, and poach for about 15 minutes or until the quinoa is cooked and the liquid is absorbed.
- Remove from heat and let it sit covered for 5 minutes
- Fluff with a chopstick and set away.
- In a large skillet, toast the olive oil over medium heat.
- Add the minced onion and cook until translucent, about 3- 4 minutes
- Add the diced garlic and cook for another nanosecond.
- Add the minced bell pepper and sludge kernels to the skillet.

- Cook for about 5 minutes, or until the vegetables are tender.
- Stir in the black sap, ground cumin, chili greasepaint, swab, and pepper.
- Cook for another 2- 3 minutes to toast through.
- Add the cooked quinoa to the skillet and mix well with the vegetable-bean admixture.
- Cook for more minutes to allow the flavors to mix together.
- Remove the skillet from heat and squeeze the lime juice over the quinoa admixture. Stir to combine.
- Serve the Mexican-
-
- Inspired Quinoa Bowl briskly, garnished with diced fresh cilantro and avocado slices. Serve with salsa on the side, and fresh condiments if asked .
- Enjoy your vibrant and nutritious Mexican-inspired quinoa bowl! Let me know if you have any questions or need further assistance.

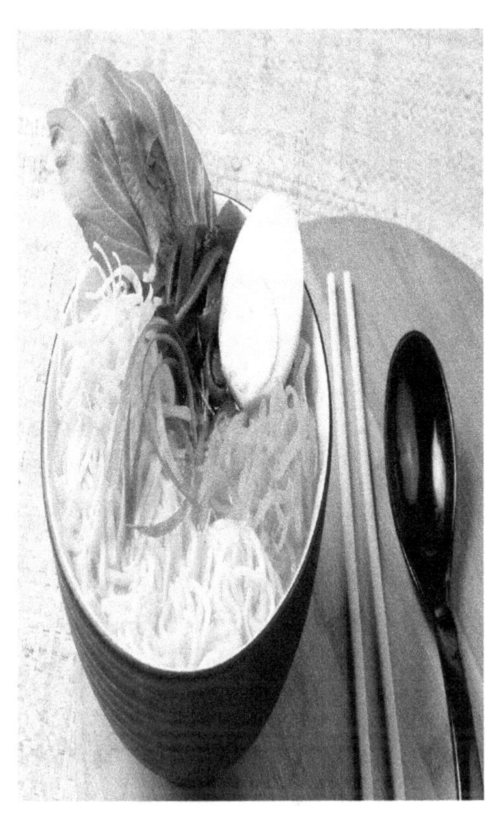

CHAPTER EIGHT

Comforting Casseroles And Bakes

Baked Ziti with Spinach and Ricotta

Ingredients

- 1 pound ziti pasta
- 2 mugs ricotta rubbish
- 2 mugs marinara sauce
- 2 mugs fresh spinach,
- minced mug mozzarella cheese
- 2 mug Parmesan cheese, grated egg
- 2 cloves garlic,
- minced tar and pepper to taste
- Olive oil

Instructions

- Preheat the rotisserie to 375 °F(190 °C).
- Grease a 9x13 inch baking dish with olive oil
- Cook the ziti pasta according to package instructions until al dente.
- Drain and set away.

- In a large bowl, combine the ricotta rubbish, egg, garlic, spinach, tar, and pepper.
- Mix well.
- In the set baking dish, spread a thin estate of marinara sauce.
- Subcaste half of the cooked ziti over the sauce. Spread the ricotta and spinach admixture over the pasta
- . Add another pinch of marinara sauce
- . Subcaste the remaining ziti on top.
- Spread the remaining marinara sauce over the top. Sprinkle with mozzarella and Parmesan crapola Cover with counter and sear for 20 beats.
- Remove the counter and sear for an fresh 10- 15 beats, until the it is melted and bubbly.
- Let it cool for a numerous beats before serving.

Vegetable and Lentil Shepherd's Pie

Ingredients

- 1 mug green or brown lentils, irrigated
- mugs vegetable broth
- 2 soupspoons olive oil

- 1 onion, minced carrots, diced celery stalks, diced cloves garlic,
- minced mug mushrooms,
- sliced mug concrete peas
- 1 tablespoon tomato paste
- 1 tablespoon soy sauce
- 1 teaspoon thyme
- 1 teaspoon rosemary tar and pepper to taste 4 mugs mashed potatoes(set singly)

Instructions

- Preheat the rotisserie to 400 °F(200 °C).
- In a pot, bring the lentils and vegetable broth to a papule.
- Reduce heat and simmer for about 20- 25 beats, until lentils are tender.
- Drain and set away.
- In a large skillet, toast the olive oil over medium heat.
- Add the onion, carrots, and celery.
- Cook until softened, about 5- 7 beats.
- Add the garlic and mushrooms, and cook for another 5 beats.
- Stir in the cooked lentils, peas, tomato paste, soy sauce, thyme, rosemary, tar, and pepper

- . Cook for another 5 beats, allowing flavors to blend.
- Transfer the vegetable and lentil together to a baking dish.
- Spread the mashed potatoes inversely over the top. sear for 20- 25 beats, until the top is golden brown. Let it rest for a numerous beats before serving.

Butternut Squash and Kale Lasagna

Ingredients

- 1 butternut squash,
- peeled and sliced bunch kale, stems
- removed and minced lasagna pates
- 2 mugs ricotta
- 2 mugs marinara sauce
- 1 mug mozzarella paste,
- 2 mug Parmesan grated egg tar and pepper to taste
- Olive oill for greasing

Instructions

- Preheat the rotisserie to 375 °F(190 °C).

- Grease a 9x13 inch baking dish with olive oil
- . Cook the lasagna pates according to package instructions.
- Drain and set away.
- In a large bowl, combine the ricotta rubbish, egg, tar, and pepper.
- Mix well.
- In the set baking dish, spread a thin of marinara sauce.
- Subcaste three lasagna pates over the sauce. Spread half of the ricotta admixture over the pates. Subcaste half of the butternut squash slices and minced kale over the ricotta.
- Add another taste of marinara sauce.
- Repeat the layers with remaining pates, ricotta, butternut squash, kale, and marinara sauce. Sprinkle with mozzarella and Parmesan crapola Cover with counter and sear for 30 beats.
- Remove the counter and sear for an fresh 10- 15 beats, until it is melted and bubbly.
- Let it cool for a numerous beats before serving.

Cheesy Broccoli and Rice Casserole

Ingredients

- 2 mugs cooked rice
- 4 mugs broccoli arrangements
- 1 mug cheddar , tattered
- 2 mug Parmesan grated mug milk
- 2 soupspoons adulation
- 2 soupspoons flour
- 1 small onion,
- minced cloves garlic,
- minced tar and pepper to taste Olive oil

Instructions

- Preheat the rotisserie to 350 °F(175 °C).
- Grease a 9x13 inch baking dish with olive oil
- Cook the broccoli in boiling water for 3- 4 beats until just tender.
- Drain and set away.
- In a saucepan, melt the adulation over medium heat.
- Add the onion and garlic, cooking until softened. Stir in the flour and cook for 1- 2 beats.
- Gradually add the milk, whisking until smooth and thickened.

- Stir in the cheddar rubber tar, and pepper until melted and combined.
- In a large bowl, combine the cooked rice, broccoli, and sauce.
- Mix well.
- Transfer the mixture to the set baking dish. Sprinkle with Parmesan together
- . sear for 20- 25 beats, until the top is golden and bubbly.
- Let it cool for a numerous beats before serving. Enjoy these succulent and comforting fashion.

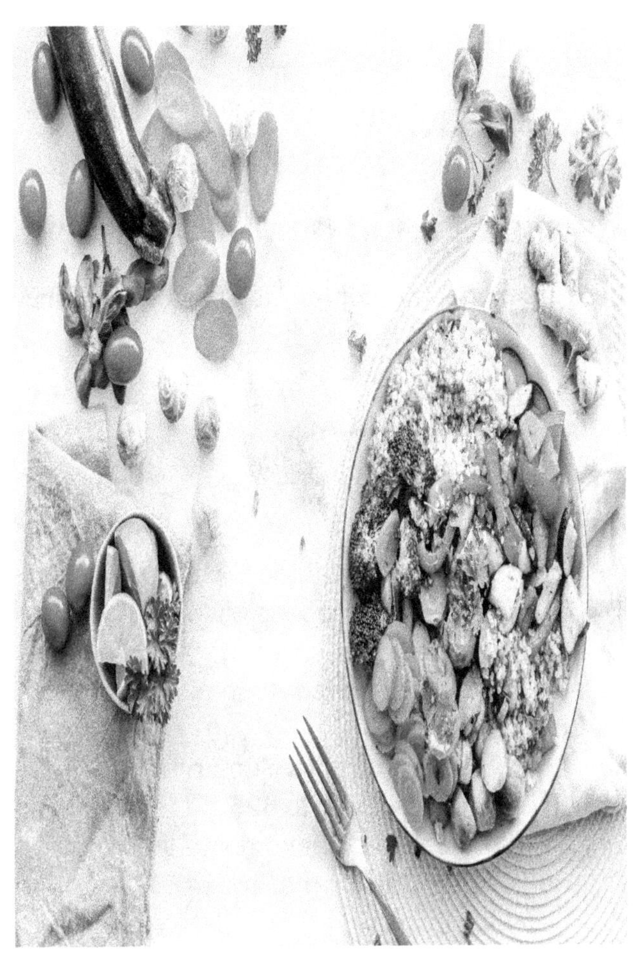

CHAPTER NINE

Side dishes and accompaniment

These are the recipes for the side dishes mentioned earlier:

Garlic Roasted Potatoes

Ingredients

- 2 pounds small potatoes, bestowed cloves garlic, diced soupspoons olive oil
- 1 tablespoon dried thyme
- 1 tablespoon dried rosemary swab and pepper to taste
- Fresh parsley, diced(voluntary, for trim)
- Preheat the roaster to 425 °F(220 °C).
- In a large coliseum, combine the potatoes, garlic, olive oil, thyme, rosemary, salt, and pepper.
- Toss until the potatoes are unevenly carpeted. Spread the potatoes in a single subcaste on a baking distance.
- rally in the preheated roaster for 25- 30 minutes turning half through, until the potatoes are golden brown and crisp.
- Garnish with fresh parsley before serving, if asked

Sautéed Green sap with Almonds

Ingredients

- 1 pound fresh green sap,
- trimmed soupspoons olive oil
- 3 cloves garlic, diced
- 4 mug sliced almonds swab and pepper to taste Lemon zest(voluntary, for trim)
- Instructions
- Blanch the green sap in boiling water for 3- 4 minutes, until tender-crisp.
- Drain and set away.
- In a large skillet, toast the olive oil over medium heat.
- Add the garlic and sauté for 1- 2 minutes until ambrosial.
- Add the bleached green sap and sauté for 5- 7 minutes, until tender.
- Stir in the sliced almonds and cook for another 2- 3 minutes, until the almonds are smoothly heated. Season with swab and pepper to taste.
- Garnish with bomb tang before serving, if asked .

Quinoa Pilaf with Dried Cranberries

Ingredients

- 1 mug quinoa, irrigated mugs vegetable broth mug dried
- cranberries mug sliced almonds
- 1 small onion,
- finely diced cloves garlic
- , diced soupspoons
- olive oil
- swab and pepper to taste
- Fresh parsley, diced(voluntary, for trim)
- Instructions
- In a medium saucepan, toast the olive oil over medium heat.
- Add the onion and garlic and sauté until softened, about 3- 4 minutes
- Add the quinoa and cook for 1- 2 minutes stirring constantly.
- Pour in the vegetable broth and bring to a pustule. Reduce the heat to low, cover, and poach for 15- 20 minutes until the quinoa is cooked and the liquid is absorbed.
- Stir in the dried cranberries and sliced almonds. Season with swab and pepper to taste.
- Garnish with fresh parsley before serving, if asked .

Delicate Mashed Cauliflower

Ingredients

- 1 large head cauliflower, cut into boutonnieres soup spoons adulation mug heavy cream
- 3 cloves garlic, diced / 4 mug Parmesan
- grated swab and pepper to taste Fresh chives, diced(voluntary, for trim)
- Instructions
- Bring a large pot of interspersed water to a pustule.
- Add the cauliflower boutonnieres and cook until veritably tender, about 10- 12 minutes.
- Drain well.
- In the same pot, melt the adulation over medium heat. Add the garlic and sauté for 1- 2 minutes until ambrosial.
- Return the cauliflower to the pot and crush until smooth(you can also use a food processor or absorption blender for a smoother texture).
- Stir in the heavy cream and Parmesan
- Mix until well combined.
- Season with swab and pepper to taste.
- Garnish with fresh chives before serving, if asked . Enjoy these succulent and healthy

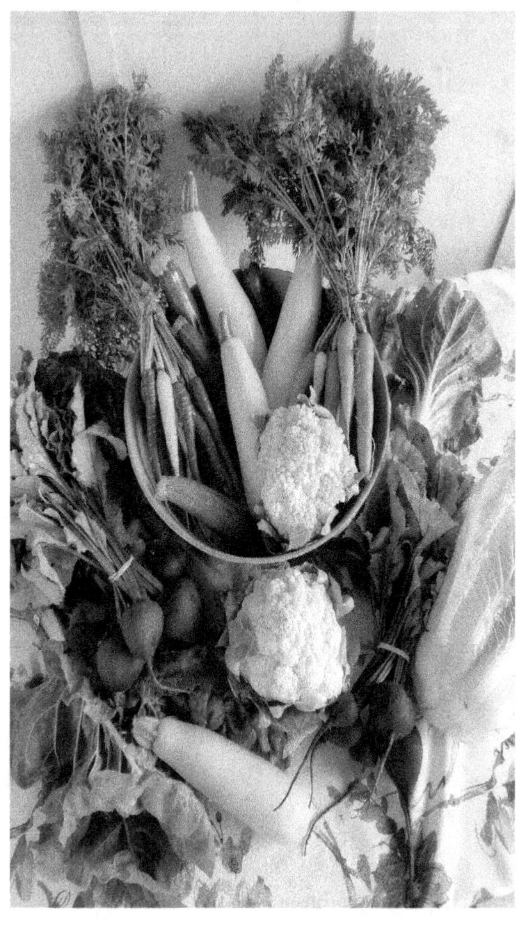

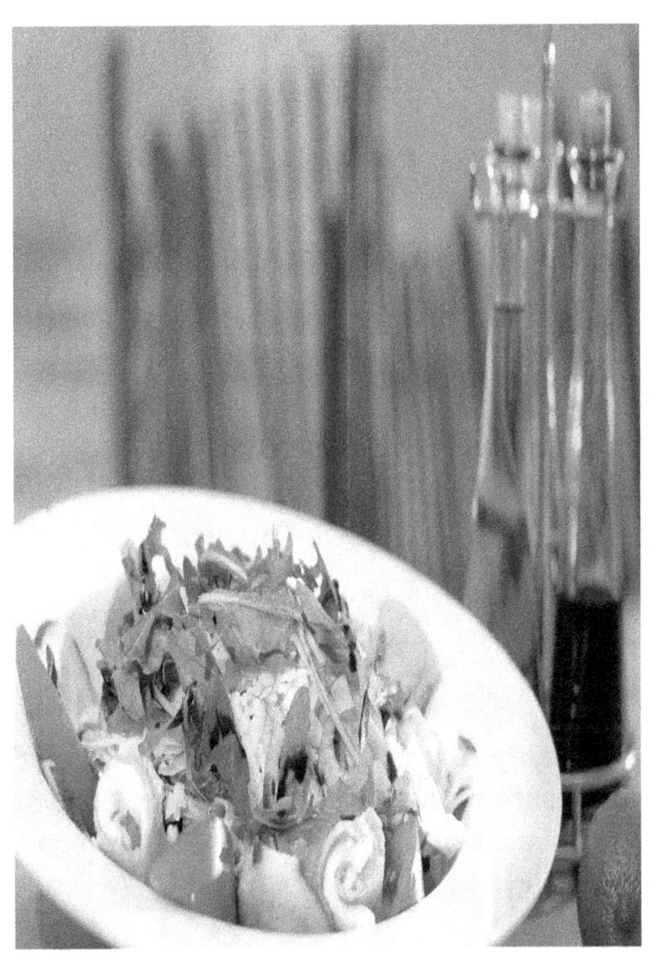

CHAPTER TEN

DECADENT DESSERTS

Chocolate Avocado Mousse

A rich and delicate chocolate mousse made with avocado.
Vegan Banana Bread with Walnuts : A wettish and scrumptious banana bread with walnuts.

Berry Crisp with Oat Topping

A sweet and crunchy berry crisp with an oat topping. Coconut Rice Pudding with Mango Slices

A creamy coconut rice pudding topped with fresh mango slices. These goodies sound succulent and healthy! These are some tense fashions for each Chocolate Avocado Scum

Ingredients

- 2 ripe avocados mug cocoa greasepaint mug maple saccharinity
- 1 tsp vanilla prize Pinch of swab

Instructions

- Mix all ingredients in a food processor until smooth.
- Chill in the refrigerator for at least 30 minutes before serving.

Vegan Banana Bread with Walnuts

Ingredients

- 3 ripe bananas, mashed
- 3 mug coconut oil melted
- 2 mug maple saccharinity
- 1 tsp vanilla excerpt mugs
- whole wheat flour
- 1 tsp baking soda pop tsp swab mug diced walnuts

Instructions

- Preheat the roaster to 350 °F(175 °C).
- Grease a loaf visage.
- Mix mashed bananas, coconut oil, maple saccharinity, and vanilla.
- In a separate coliseum, blend flour, incinerating soda pop, and swab.
- Combine wet and dry constituents, also fold in walnuts.

- Pour batter into the loaf visage and singe for 50- 60 minutes.

Berry Crisp with Oat Beating

Ingredients

- 4 mugs mixed berries(fresh or frozen) mug sugar(voluntary)
- 1 tbsp bomb juice
- 1 mug rolled oats mug almond flour mug coconut oil melted
- 4 mug maple saccharinity
- 1 tsp cinnamon

Instructions

- Preheat roaster to 375 °F(190 °C).
- Grease a baking dish.
- Mix berries, sugar(if using), and bomb juice, also spread in the dish.
- Combine oats, almond flour, coconut oil, maple saccharinity, and cinnamon.
- Sprinkle over berries.
- Singe for 30- 35 minutes until beating is golden.

Coconut Rice Pudding with Mango Slices

Ingredients

- 1 mug jasmine rice
- 2 mugs coconut milk
- 1 mug water mug sugar
- 1 tsp vanilla excerpt
- Fresh mango slices

Instructions

- Combine rice, coconut milk, water, and sugar in a pot. Bring to a pustule.
- Reduce heat and poach, stirring sometimes, until rice is tender and mixture is delicate(about 20- 25 minuites).
- Stir in vanilla excerpt.
- Serve warm or stupefied with fresh mango slices on top. Enjoy these pleasurable and nutritional goodies

CHAPTER ELEVEN

Beverages and refreshments

Iced Matcha Latte

Ingredients

- 1 tablespoon matcha greasepaint
- 2 soupspoons hot water
- 1 mug milk(dairy or factory- grounded)
- 1- 2 ladles sweetener(like honey, maple saccharinity, or sugar)
- , voluntary Ice cells
- Instructions
- In a small coliseum, whisk the matcha greasepaint with the hot water until it forms a smooth paste.
- Fill a glass with ice cells.
- Pour the milk over the ice.
- Add the matcha admixture to the glass and stir well to combine.
- Candy to taste if asked .

Berry Smoothie with Spinach

Ingredients

- 1 mug mixed berries(fresh or frozen)
- 1 sprinkle fresh spinach leaves
- 1 banana
- 1 mug unsweetened almond milk(or any milk of choice)
- 1 teaspoon chia seeds(voluntary)
- 1 tablespoon honey or maple saccharinity(voluntary)
- Instructions
- Combine all ingredients in a blender.
- mix until smooth and delicate.
- Taste and add sweetener if demanded
- . Pour into a glass and enjoy incontinently.

Herbal Infusions and Tea Blends

Ingredients

- 1. Mint and Ginger Tea Fresh mint leaves Fresh gusto slices Honey(voluntary)
- Hot water

Instructions

- In a teapot or mug, add a sprinkle of mint leaves and a many slices of fresh gusto.
- Pour hot water over the sauces and let it steep for 5- 10 minutes
- Strain and candy with honey if asked .
- Chamomile and Lavender Tea:
- Dried chamomile flowers Dried lavender kids Honey(voluntary)
- Hot water

Instructions

- In a teapot or mug, add 1 tablespoon of dried chamomile flowers and1/2 tablespoon of dried lavender kids.
- Pour hot water over the flowers and let it steep for 5- 7 minutes.
- Strain and candy with honey if asked .
- Lemon Balm and Lemon Verbena Tea Fresh
- bomb attar leaves Fresh bomb verbena leaves Honey(voluntary)
- Hot water

Instructions

- In a teapot or mug, add a sprinkle of bomb attar and bomb verbena leaves.
- Pour hot water over the leaves and let it steep for 5- 10 minutes
- Strain and candy with honey if asked . Feel free to acclimate the component amounts to suit your taste preferences. Enjoy your stimulating and nutritional Lemon verbena tea drinks

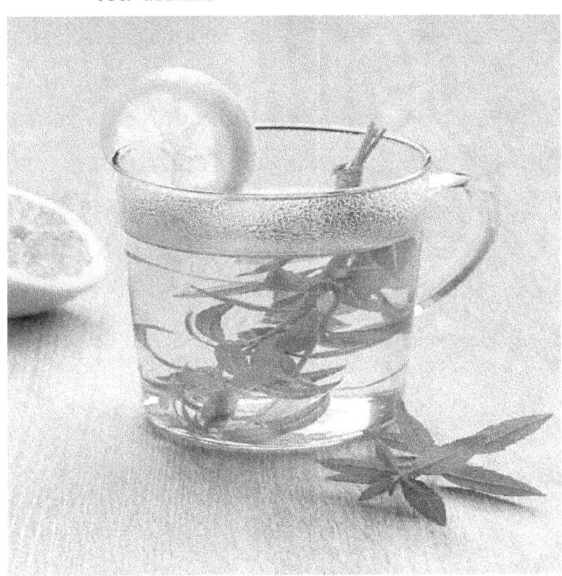

CHAPTER TWELVE

Conclusion

Incorporating the Vegetarian Cookbook for Beginners 2024 into your collection is an investment in your health, your culinary skills, and the environment. Its comprehensive approach, combining nutritional guidance, ease of use, variety, and practical tips, makes it an indispensable resource for anyone looking to adopt a vegetarian lifestyle. Whether you're a seasoned cook or a kitchen novice, this cookbook will guide you on a rewarding journey towards vibrant health and sustainable living. By making it a part of your cookbook list, you are choosing a path of culinary exploration, enhanced well-being, and a positive impact on the planet.

Additional Resources For Further Readings

Further Reading and Cookbooks on Vegetarian Cooking
"Plenty" by Yotam Ottolenghi - A celebrated cookbook featuring vibrant and inventive vegetarian recipes.
"The Moosewood Cookbook" by Mollie Katzen - A classic that has inspired generations of vegetarian cooks with its accessible and delicious recipes.
"Vegetable Kingdom" by Bryant Terry - Focuses on plant-based cooking with a cultural perspective, featuring a range of flavorful dishes.

"How to Cook Everything Vegetarian" by Mark Bittman - A comprehensive guide that covers a wide variety of vegetarian recipes.
"Isa Does It" by Isa Chandra Moskowitz - Offers easy-to-make, delicious vegan recipes for everyday cooking.

"The First Mess Cookbook" by Laura Wright -
Features seasonal and wholesome plant-based
recipes with beautiful photography.

Online Communities and Websites
Vegetarian Times - Offers recipes, articles, and
tips for vegetarian and vegan cooking.
Oh She Glows - Angela Liddon's website with a
plethora of plant-based recipes and meal ideas.

Minimalist Baker - Features simple, quick, and
delicious vegetarian and vegan recipes.
Veganuary - Provides resources, recipes, and a
supportive community for those
exploring a plant-based diet.

HappyCow - An online community and resource
for finding vegetarian and vegan restaurants
worldwide.

Reddit: r/vegetarian - A forum for sharing
recipes, tips, and experiences related to
vegetarianism.
 Cooking Classes and Workshops

Local Community Centers and Adult Education
Programs - Many local community centers offer
cooking classes, including vegetarian options.

Check with your local center or adult education programs for schedules.

Sur La Table - Offers cooking classes across the U.S., including vegetarian-specific sessions.

The Natural Gourmet Institute - Specializes in health-supportive culinary education, offering vegetarian and vegan courses.
Rouxbe Online Culinary School - Provides online cooking courses, including
plant-based cooking.

Forks Over Knives Cooking Course - An online course focusing on whole-food, plant-based cooking.

Local Health Food Stores and Co-ops - Many health food stores and co-ops host

cooking classes and workshops. Find out what activities are coming up at your neighborhood store.

These resources should provide a solid foundation for exploring vegetarian cooking, connecting with like-minded individuals, and expanding your culinary skills.

www.ingramcontent.com/pod-product-compliance
Lightning Source LLC
Chambersburg PA
CBHW071224260726
48653CB00042B/2080